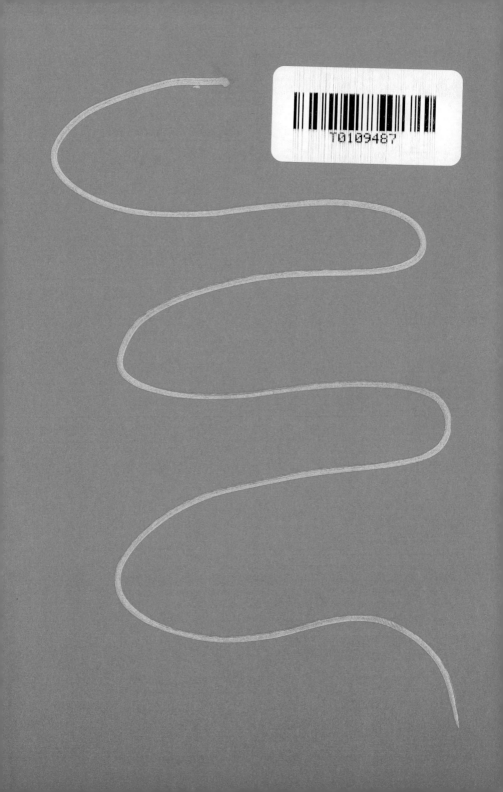

MOM HACKS

MOM
HACKS

200 LIFESAVING PARENTING TIPS
AND TRICKS FROM SUPER MOMS

HOPE COMERFORD

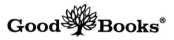

Good Books®

New York, New York

Good Books books may be purchased in bulk at special discounts for sales promotion, corporate gifts, fund-raising, or educational purposes. Special editions can also be created to specifications. For details, contact the Special Sales Department, Skyhorse Publishing, 307 West 36th Street, 11th Floor, New York, NY 10018 or info@skyhorsepublishing.com.

Good Books is an imprint of Skyhorse Publishing, Inc.®, a Delaware corporation.

Visit our website at www.goodbooks.com.

10 9 8 7 6 5 4 3 2 1

Library of Congress Cataloging-in-Publication Data is available on file.

Cover design by Qualcom
Cover photo credit iStock

Print ISBN: 978-1-68099-441-4
Ebook ISBN: 978-1-68099-439-1

Printed in China

CONTENTS

INTRODUCTION

♥

Being a mom is the most fulfilling, yet draining, job you'll ever have.

However, I know you wouldn't change it for the world!

But time is (always) of the essence, and finding a balance between work, shuttling the kids back and forth, making appointments and travel plans, grocery shopping, meal prepping, etc., is SO hard to do.

You know that saying "It takes a village"? Well, it's my motto. Doing this "mom thing" alone is near impossible, but I find momming becomes so much easier when you reach out to other moms for their advice, expertise, and hacks!

This book is FULL of advice from moms (and dads!) just like you! Even my own mom sent her amazing tips my way to share with you! This is a great book to keep on your e-reader, coffee table, or—let's face it—the back of your toilet (because you know the bathroom is the only place where you get some time alone!).

When you're in a conundrum, open up this book and find a solution! Always remember: you are not alone. We've got your back!

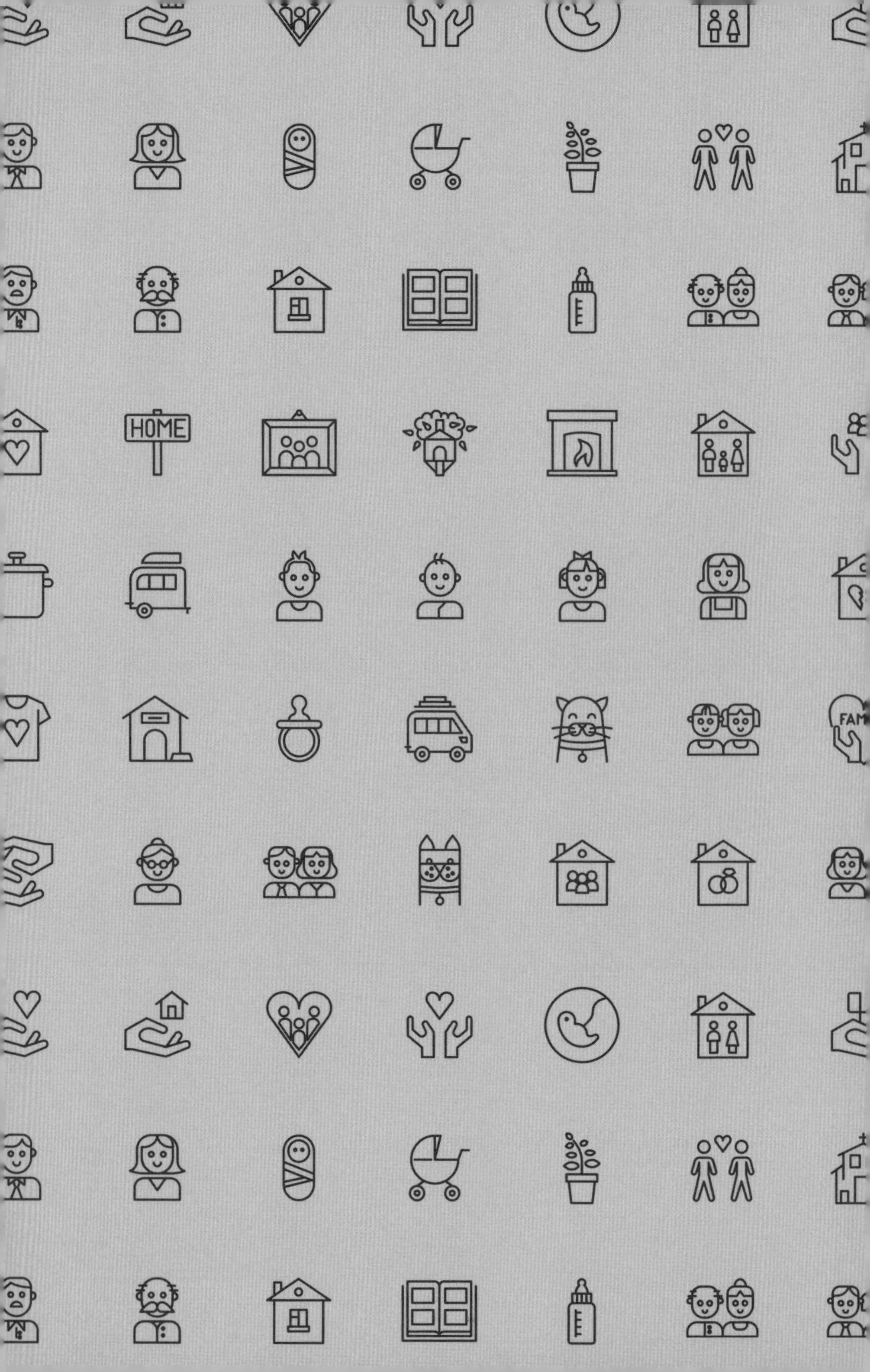
HOME

KID AND FAMILY HACKS

♥

Is your morning routine in shambles? Are your kids CONSTANTLY asking you to get them their snacks? Does the laundry sock monster keep eating your socks? Are your kids melting down in the store? The following chapter has hacks for all these things and so much more!

HACK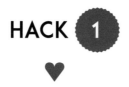

♥

"Keep a special shelf and area in your fridge for just kids' snacks, that way they know they can always go there to get a snack. It also gives you the opportunity to determine what you want them eating as snacks."

♥

—ALICIA BALL, SOUTHGATE, MI

HACK  2

♥

"Keep bowls and glasses within kids' reach so they can help themselves."

♥

—Natalie Trombley,
Rochester Hills, MI

HACK 3

♥

"Clear a big spot in your freezer, and set aside one day each month to prepare lunch items if your kids take their lunches to school every day. Lunch meat sandwiches on hamburger buns, peanut butter and jelly, grapes, berries, carrots . . . there are many 'lunchbox friendly' foods that freeze well. This has saved me a ridiculous amount of time in the hustle and bustle of the morning. Each type of item has its own container, and even the kids can reach in and pack their own. You don't even need an ice pack; put it in frozen and it IS its own ice pack. It'll still be cold at lunch time!"

♥

—LUANN EDWARDS,
WILMINGTON, OH

HACK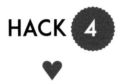

♥

"Pack your lunches for the next day the night before. If your kids are old enough, have them make up their lunches. Put everything in their lunch boxes and store in the fridge for a stress-free morning."

♥

—HEATHER S., KANSAS CITY, KS

HACK

♥

"My youngest is now a freshman in high school, and since his first day of kindergarten, he has used an alarm clock to get up for school. In the beginning, we put the clock on his dresser, so he would get up to turn it off! No snooze! I know it seems fun to go wake them up when they are young, but there is nothing worse than waking up a teen forty-seven times in the morning! He now uses it, all year, for sports, church, anything he has going on!"

♥

—Kara Dimino, Milton, GA

HACK

♥

"I would decorate a Febreze bottle and write MONSTER SPRAY on it, spray the room, and no more scary things in the room!"

♥

—Sally Tredinnick,
Wilkes-Barre, PA

HACK 7

♥

"Make any special occasion at school
even more special by adding a face to
a plastic or paper bag that holds their
treats for their special day. Also, if
someone in their class has food allergies
and can't eat the treats, provide pencils
and erasers in there, too!"

♥

—MARY LADD, LAKE ORION, MI

HACK 8

♥

"Before bed, help kids pick out clothes for the next day. This helps with the struggle of 'what will I wear today?'"

♥

—Jill Kovach, Cumming, GA

HACK

♥

"Clothes laid out, all pieces and bags packed the night before. Makes for faster exits in the morning!"

♥

—JACKIE FITCH, BURLINGTON, WI

HACK

♥

"Our kids' socks used to always disappear in the wash and I would search endlessly for the matching pair. Now I only buy six or seven sets of socks that either match or go together. This way if one (or more) sock goes missing, I still have other socks to match them with."

♥

—INGRIDA KNUEPPEL,
ROCHESTER HILLS, MI

HACK

♥

"If you only have footie PJ's that the kids are taking off when they shouldn't, just cut off the feet and then zip it up backward and the little ones won't be able to shimmy out!"

♥

—AUBREY MAYES, INDIANAPOLIS, IN

HACK 12

♥

*"Always name and date
pictures. Ten, twenty, thirty
years from now, you WILL
forget the details."*

♥

—JEAN HANSEN, BELTSVILLE, MD

♥

"Create your own paint by numbers.
Draw simple forms and break them up
into smaller shapes. Add numbers and
corresponding colors for your kids in
a key. Your children will make special,
unique pieces to display in their rooms."

♥

—MARY LADD, LAKE ORION, MI

♥

"Make a chore chart for your children.
The child that empties the dishwasher
also sets the table that day. Both jobs
can be done at once."

♥

—JOY MARTIN, RICHLAND, PA

HACK 15

♥

"I made 3 routine charts for my children.
I included a picture with each item on the list.
You can put different items on your list,
but here is ours to get you started:

Morning Routine
1. Breakfast
2. Teeth
3. Wash face & ears
4. Get dressed
5. Hair
6. Shoes

After-School Routine
1. Snuggle with Mom
2. Small healthy snack
3. Play outside
4. Homework
5. Set table
6. Practice one instrument

Evening Routine
1. Clean bedroom
2. Exercise/stretch
3. Shower/bath
4. Pajamas
5. Clothes away
6. Teeth
7. Bible Story, hymn, devotions
8. Read
9. Pray
10. Sleep"

♥

—LYNETTE BRENNEMAN, LANCASTER, PA

HACK

♥

"When your children get out the LEGO to create their amazing masterpieces, have them dump their LEGO on a bed sheet. When they have finished with their creation, cleanup is easy. Just grab the four corners of the sheet and put the whole thing in their LEGO bin. No more lost pieces for you to step on later."

♥

—CAROL EVELETH, CHEYENNE, WY

HACK

♥

"Sort children's toys in separate plastic containers with lids or in cubes. For instance, tractors in one, blocks in another. This way they don't have to dump out all the toys to find the ones they want."

♥

—JOY REIFF, MOUNT JOY, PA

HACK 18

♥

"I have the kids pick up toys three times a day; once after lunch, before naps, and again before bedtime."

♥

—JENNIFER FREED,
HARRISONBURG, VA

HACK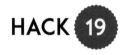

♥

"Tie a shoe caddy at the back of your car seat to hold small toys & games for your kids."

♥

—CHARLOTTE SHAFFER, EAST EARL, PA

HACKS 20-22

SUPERMOM SUGGESTIONS!

Mary Ladd, Lake Orion, MI

"Don't want to buy expensive Barbie clothes? Give the kids colored tissue or tissue paper and have them make clothes as they become the designers of unique styles!"

♥

"Have children cover their school books using plain paper bags. Decorate them with special bling decorations and leftover parts of games or puzzles to cover them."

♥

"To help children with memorization, make up crazy stories, sayings, and songs. This was how I taught my kids the state capitals."

HACK

"Keep extra paper, crayons, colored pencils, and pencils or pens handy. Keep a cup full of sharpened pencils, ready to grab to tackle that homework! This eliminates the excuse that they need to find a pencil and wasting time before starting homework. Bonus: play some classical music quietly. I found the music helps them study and focus a little better."

—BARBARA PIERCE, WURTLAND, KY

HACK  24

♥

"To organize kids' homework and school papers, I have a wall file attached to the side of the fridge. There is a folder for each child's homework and one for scrap paper."

♥

—MELISSA WENGER, DALTON, OH

HACK 25

♥

"When the kids have a lot of friends over, I give each one a different colored rubber band that I've salvaged from produce. They put the bands on our regular glasses so they can keep track of their glasses and I don't end up with every glass in my house in the sink."

♥

—JEANETTE MORGAN, NORTHBOROUGH, MA

HACK 26

♥

"Each of my five children was assigned a color. Their drinking cup was that color, their bath towel was striped that color, and their swim towel and their laundry basket was that color, too. Each was responsible for keeping these things clean."

♥

—MARJORIE B., MIDLAND, MI

HACK

"Involve your children in the cleaning process. Use nontoxic, plant-based cleaning materials such as Young Living's Thieves Cleaner or Norwex cloths so you can feel comfortable letting your little ones help you clean without putting them in harm's way. They'll be more mindful of keeping areas clean when they know what it takes to keep things clean!"

—Hope Comerford, Clinton Township, MI

HACK  28

♥

"Involve your children in the duties of the household. Make chore charts to cut out grumbling about whose turn it is to do what."

♥

—JOY MARTIN, RICHLAND, PA

HACK

"To keep young children from coming by the stove while cooking, keep them occupied and in view by having them make a picture for you using honey and feathers. The time it takes to try and get the feathers off their fingers and on the paper will give you the time to finish cooking . . . and it's hysterical to watch, too!"

—MARY LADD, LAKE ORION, MI

HACK 30

♥

"To get kids to put their shoes on the correct feet, cut a sticker in half and place it on the insides, of their shoes. They will know their shoes are on the correct feet when the sticker pieces match up."

♥

—CHARLOTTE SHAFFER,
EAST EARL, PA

HACK 31

♥

"Does your little one keep putting their shoes on the wrong feet? Put a small dot or smiley face with Sharpie in the insteps of the shoes. 'Make them touch' and the shoes will be on the correct feet. You can also put it on winter boots. Use nail polish for easy ID of the boots that all look the same at school."

♥

—LAURA BRUEDERLE, CEDARBURG, WI

HACK 32

♥

"Use frozen ketchup packets as icepacks. They are the perfect size for kids' bumps and bruises and they stay soft when frozen so they can form around any body part. They can also be used for oven burns."

♥

—Judith Manos, West Islip, NY

♥

"When our boys played baseball, we
would freeze water bottles because they
served several purposes; they would
keep food in the cooler cold, they were
great for putting on bug bites and small
injuries and keeping us cool, and of
course, for drinking."

♥

—SALLY TREDINNICK,
WILKES-BARRE, PA

HACK  34

♥

"Puppy pads work great for a bed wetter and are so much easier to change during the night!"

♥

—MARY LADD, LAKE ORION, MI

HACK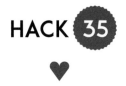

"If you don't have a bib handy for your toddler, take a dish towel and a clothespin and pin it around the neck. Tada! So easy and you have a nice big bib."

—ANGELA DIEM, DENMARK, SC

HACK 36

"During flu season, always keep
a plastic bag in your purse!
It will save your purse!"

♥

—MARY LADD, LAKE ORION, MI

HACK

♥

"For families with iPhones, learn how and utilize the ability to share calendars. It makes keeping up with everyone's schedule so much easier . . . even husbands can do it!"

♥

—ALICIA BALL, SOUTHGATE, MI

HACK 38

♥

"Use a binder clip to hold your
used toothpaste tube as you
wind down the tube."

♥

—BARBARA SHIE,
COLORADO SPRINGS, CO

HACK  39

♥

"When shopping or running errands with kids or even by yourself, pack a bag filled with granola bars, snacks, and drinks. When the urge hits, you don't have to stop to fuel the kids (or yourself), and you can eliminate excess food-buying at the store!"

♥

—MICHELE RUVOLA, VESTAL, NY

HACK

♥

"When my kids were little, the way I would prevent tantrums and meltdowns in stores was to keep sticker packets in the car and reward good behavior with stickers when we got back to the car. Any time they would start to act up, I would remind them of the stickers and they would immediately be on their best behavior."

♥

—TIFFANY LANGDON, LYNNFIELD, MA

"Make a 'Must-do' list for summer break. Make an age-appropriate list, or Bingo board with spaces filled in. Kids have to complete two to three things or get a Bingo before they can have technology."

♥

—VICKIE ZOLLER, TROY, MI

HACK

♥

"When on a beach, upon leaving, use baby powder for removing sand from the skin."

♥

—Lynn Inverso, Warrington, PA

HACKS 43-45

SUPER(GRAND)MOM SUGGESTIONS!

Theresa Eulberg, Forest Falls, CA

"When the grandbabies come over for the weekend and you don't want to chase them all over the house, confine them to one room by closing all doors to that room and getting baby gates that go up in every open entryway. Make sure that all breakables are put up, and things you don't want them touching are all put up. The baby has access to the entire room while you're sitting in that same room relaxing, with no worries about the baby running off to another room and you having to chase him or her, and no risk to their safety."

"Plastic storage bins make great containers for grandbaby supplies. When my granddaughter was a baby, I had a plastic bin under the bed that contained all of her diapering supplies; diapers, wipes, change of clothes, etc. When she would come over, I would only have to pull one box out from under the bed to change her diaper. I also keep all of her art and activity supplies in bins. When she comes over, she knows exactly where her art supplies are, and typically the first thing she says is she wants to color or play with her blocks. I can go right to the shelf where they are stored, pull down one box that has all of her crayons, markers, colored pencils, or the other container that has all of her blocks to play with. It helps to keep my house organized and neat and easy to access when the grandkids come over."

♥

"Always have a random supply of arts and crafts activities for the grandkids to do when they come over to visit. I go to the craft stores, Walmart, Target, dollar stores, and buy small to large crafts, and keep them stashed away in a closet. When the grandbaby comes over, I can give her a choice of a few different projects to do. Anything from paint supplies and painting rocks, painting on canvas, making cement stepping-stones, beads, coloring books, supplies and ingredients for baking with Grandma, and lots of books to read. My granddaughter loves to visit and is always excited to find out what the craft will be that day."

♥

HACK 46

♥

"A small plastic pool just outside the kitchen will keep a new crawling baby from danger."

♥

—MARY LADD, LAKE ORION, MI

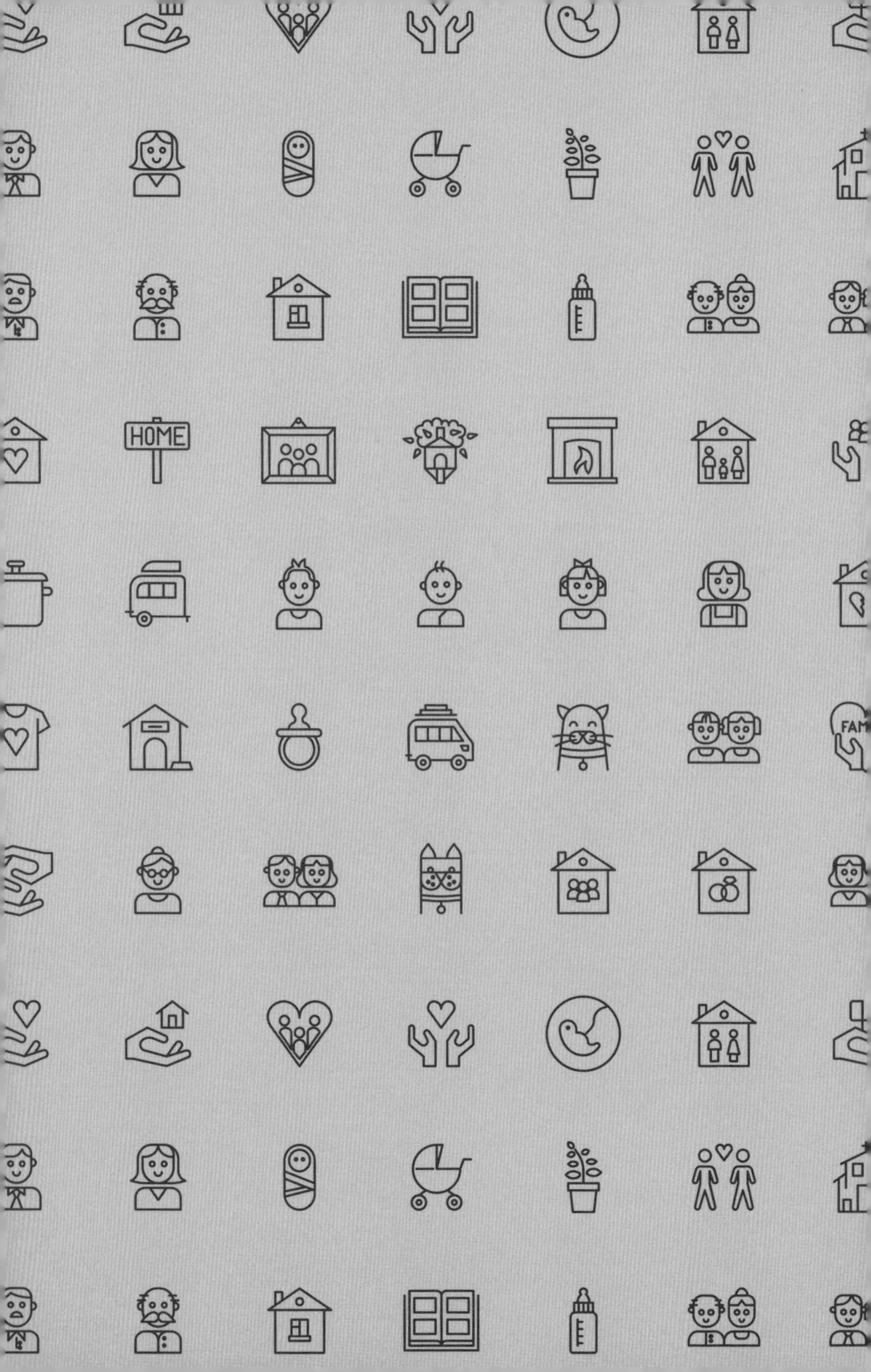
HOME

COOKING HACKS

♥

We all have that friend: Supermom. You know, the one who seems to have it ALL together? She grocery shops like a pro, then has a beautiful dinner on the table each night that her kids eat EVERY bite of?! The following chapter has some ideas when it comes to cooking and food to help YOUR inner Supermom show up to the game!

HACK 47

♥

"Do meal prep and/or freezer workshops.
I suggest Wildtree, but any way is fine.
Invite friends over for snacks and wine
while you prep. You're setting yourself up
with ten to twelve meals. Easy-peasy."

♥

—VICKIE ZOLLER, TROY, MI

HACK  48

♥

"As a mom of four, I was always battling picky eaters and trying to come up with dinner ideas that would make everyone happy. I sat down with all of the children and asked them to plan their *favorite* meal; main dish and sides (and dessert if they chose). Each one usually had at least two favorite meals they wrote down (or had me write). This gave me a full week's worth of meal plans and my picky eaters were willing to eat what their sibs had planned, knowing that the next meal would be one that they had planned."

♥

—AVONELLE SOLLARS, ALBANY, OH

HACK 49

♥

"Let your kids help plan, prepare, and clean up dinner! My kids eat a lot better if they have a say in what we have and they all enjoy getting cooking time with Mom!"

♥

—BARBARA PIERCE, WURTLAND, KY

HACK 50

♥

"I always had my kids help prepare the food (scrub veggies, measure ingredients, even cut as they got older). They added the ingredients and stirred during preparation. When they saw what went into a dish, they were more willing to try the new foods. My children are grown now and all four LOVE to cook. One is a chef at a local restaurant."

♥

—AVONELLE SOLLARS, ALBANY, OH

HACK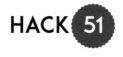

♥

"Forgot to take meat out of the freezer? Purchase a rotisserie chicken! Shred it up and you can have salad, tacos, quesadillas, or fajitas."

♥

—Cathy McIntosh,
Chesterfield Township, MI

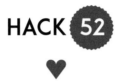

HACK 52

"I make double batches of soups, stews, sauces, and chilis and freeze them in quart mason jars with reusable plastic lids. I use masking tape to label the lids. I've even been known to do this with smoothies and then pull them out the night before so they thaw in the fridge for my drive to work."

—JEANETTE MORGAN, NORTHBOROUGH, MA

HACK

"When making Sunday dinner, cook
two meats. The oven is on anyway!
You will have one main dish cooked,
then reheat with two sides [the next day],
and dinner is done."

♥

—VICKI AKINS,
SHELBY TOWNSHIP, MI

HACK  54

♥

"Cook once, eat three times! Cook large batches of things that can be eaten different ways; roast beef one night, shredded beef tacos next night, then BBQ beef sandwiches the next night. Big batch of soup? Serve it with cheese bread, then the next night with salad, and the next night with grilled cheese!"

♥

—Carolyn Dougharty,
San Diego, CA

HACK  55

♥

"Due to busy schedules, for both kids and parents, everyone is eating at different times. I will cook a batch of seasoned ground beef so people can make tacos, nachos, or quesadillas. I also do this with pasta. I make a pot of pasta, then people can add sauce, veggies, or butter when they want to eat."

♥

—Kristin Lupo, Stratford, CT

HACK  56

♥

"Try to make something ahead of time. My kids love being able to go to the freezer and get something out they can pop in the microwave for a quick snack or meal."

♥

—BARBARA PIERCE, WURTLAND, KY

HACK  57

♥

"Make breakfast burritos in advance for hot breakfast in four minutes. We use eggs, bacon, hash browns, and cheese. Cook ingredients and put in flour tortillas. Make about thirty at a time. Put them in sandwich bags and then in gallon freezer bags. We microwave for four minutes."

♥

—ANGELA NYLUND, BORING, OR

HACK 58

♥

"Make egg sandwiches and wraps in
large quantities. Wrap in foil and
freeze for an easy breakfast."

♥

—JOY MARTIN, RICHLAND, PA

HACK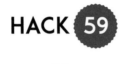

"Make double batches of weekend breakfasts (waffles, pancakes, etc.) and freeze for quick and easy breakfasts during the week."

—JACKIE FITCH, BURLINGTON, WI

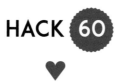

HACK 60

♥

"Bake pancake batter on a jelly roll pan.
It cuts the stress of hungry children
waiting while you fry."

♥

—JOY MARTIN, RICHLAND, PA

HACK

♥

"When frying bacon, use a stockpot instead of a frying pan. Keeps the stove cleaner and won't splash hot grease on any little ones who might be walking by."

♥

—THERESA TOMPOROWSKI,
MERIDEN, CT

HACK 62

"I never fry bacon on the stovetop anymore. I throw it on a cookie sheet in the oven and forget it until it's time to take out: 15 mins at 400 degrees. Perfect every time. No mess!"

—LORI STILTS, ATASCADERO, CA

HACK

♥

"Frozen chopped onions! Total life
and time saver. Instead of crying over
chopping onions, we buy bags of pre-
diced onions in the frozen foods section.
We may pay a tiny bit more, but it saves
me time and aggravation."

♥

—SHANI BELL, PHOENIX, AZ

HACK 64

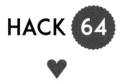

♥

"When freezing onion, lay them in a single layer in freezer, then when frozen, put them in a bucket in the freezer. Then you can scoop out as many as you want."

♥

—JOY REIFF, MOUNT JOY, PA

HACK 65

♥

"I love using fresh ingredients, but I don't always have some on hand. So, I freeze them. It may not be super fresh, but I still get the flavor. I store cut up ginger pieces in the freezer and it's easy to pop out and grate. If I grate a lemon or lime for zest, I cut the rest of the lemon into quarters and freeze. I store frozen garlic the same way; break out from the whole bulb, peel, and freeze. I also store leftover tomato paste and homemade pesto in small silicone ice cube trays from Pampered Chef. Pop them out when ready, let thaw while you're cooking, and pop them in with your other ingredients."

♥

—CARRI FAICH, CHATHAM, NJ

HACK 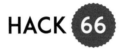 66

♥

"Save leftovers (meat and vegetables) in the freezer for soup stock."

♥

—Vicki Akins, Shelby Township, MI

HACK  67

♥

"Buy things on sale and freeze,
or to stock up your pantry."

♥

—CAROLYN DOUGHARTY,
SAN DIEGO, CA

HACK 68

"Buy ground beef on sale. Buy in bulk and cook it all down so you have cooked ground beef. Lay parchment on a cookie/baking sheet and spread the cooked ground beef on the tray. Freeze overnight and then pour the crumbles into a Ziploc. I usually measure out before I store. When you're ready to use, simply dump out into a pan with a tablespoon of water and let it warm up. Add your favorite sauce or flavoring!"

—CARRI FAICH, CHATHAM, NJ

♥

"Buy ground meat in bulk and cook it all. Freeze in one-pound portions. One pound of uncooked meat is equal to 2.5 cups cooked. Great to have on hand for quick and easy meals—tacos, sloppy joes, spaghetti, etc."

♥

—Jackie Fitch, Burlington, WI

HACK  70

♥

"I, like many of you, buy ground beef in bulk. Do you find yourself running out of room in your freezer? I put my portions in freezer bags and roll them with my rolling pin till they are flat. They are so much easier to store and take up less room."

♥

—ELLEN WORTHEN, TIPP CITY, OH

HACK

♥

"Cook a bunch of chicken, dice, and measure it out in 2 or 4 cups into a Ziploc bag and freeze. This is so handy to have ready when you want cooked chicken for a casserole or soup."

♥

—JOY MARTIN, RICHLAND, PA

HACK  72

♥

"You can sub applesauce (unsweetened is best) for oil or butter in any baking recipe! Cut those calories and feel a little less guilty while you indulge in some delicious baked goods."

♥

—Hope Comerford, Clinton Township, MI

HACK

♥

"I always end up with leftover tomato
sauce. I measure and pour the rest
into small Ziploc bags and freeze flat.
Make sure to write the brand and flavor.
Eventually I have enough bags for a meal.
To thaw, take out and place on counter,
or just dump into a microwave-safe bowl
and warm up a little."

♥

—CARRI FAICH, CHATHAM, NJ

HACK

♥

"We all have busy schedules, so on your day off or when veggies are on sale, stock up. I often freeze veggies, which speeds up food prep later on. I chop onions, slice or chop peppers, shred carrots and potatoes, etc."

♥

—Anita Troyer, Fairview, MI

HACK  75

♥

"Want to teach your kids bake but don't want to eat cookies every day? Have them bake dog treats instead!"

♥

—Mary Ladd, Lake Orion, MI

HACK  76

♥

"Need to cool down soup or stew quickly? Stir some frozen veggies into the meal instead of ice cubes. Cools it down fast and is a good way to sneak in some more veggies."

♥

—LAURA BRUEDERLE,
CEDARBURG, WI

HACK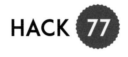

♥

"Put soggy fries from fast food or carry out box into the Air Fryer on 400 degrees for 10 minutes to make them crispy again."

♥

—Jo Ann Diffenderfer, Perry, MO

HACK

♥

"To ice whoopie pies, fill an icing bag with the filling and use a big round tip. Squeeze icing onto one cookie and then top with the other cookie. So easy and takes less time than icing with a knife."

♥

—ANGELA DIEM, DENMARK, SC

HACK  79

♥

"To smooth out sticky brownie or bar batter, use a smooth, curved spatula!"

♥

—Angela Diem, Denmark, SC

HACK 80

♥

"I love chocolate chip cookies. Don't really care for the mixing and such of the process. Two days ago, I decided to try making a HUGE batch then spread the dough on a parchment-lined baking sheet (I used one of the huge ones usually used for making jelly roll cake.) I put it in the fridge overnight. The next day, I took the pan from the fridge and removed the parchment paper with cookie dough out of the pan and onto my counter. I cut the dough the size I wanted in strips, then cut the other way making squares. I split the squares onto two parchment-lined cookie sheets so the squares didn't touch, re-using the first parchment paper and put back in the fridge to re-harden for an hour. I then removed the squares and put into plastic containers. I froze some for later use and put one container into the fridge. I made a few cookies today and they taste as good as if I had just freshly made the dough. Now I can make cookies whenever the mood strikes."

♥

—Linda Dobson, McMinnville, OR

HACK

♥

"Instead of making s'mores with the traditional graham crackers, chocolate candy bar, and roasted marshmallow, buy the fudge-covered (chocolate-covered) graham cookies and put your roasted marshmallow between two cookies. No more waiting for the chocolate to melt."

♥

—CAROL EVELETH, CHEYENNE, WY

HACK 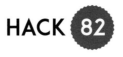 82

♥

"To keep a cake moist, fill a shot class with water and put it on the plate before covering leftover cake."

♥

—Barbara Nolan, Pleasant Valley, NY

HACK  83

♥

"To keep lettuce crisp, I store it in a gallon Ziploc bag with paper towels lying against the inside of the bag."

♥

—MELISSA WENGER, DALTON, OH

HACK 84

"To keep sliced apples from browning, make a solution of ½ teaspoon Kosher salt with 1 cup water. Soak slices for 10 minutes. Drain. You can rinse if desired to remove the small amount of salt flavor, but it won't be that strong. Keep slices in airtight container for several days."

—BARBARA NOLAN,
PLEASANT VALLEY, NY

HACK  85

♥

"An easy way to keep apples from browning is to add a bit of citrus to them. I usually add a touch of lemon or lime juice to my apples and either stir, or shake, depending on what I'm storing them in. Not only do they not brown, but it really brings out the flavor of the apple."

♥

—HOPE COMERFORD,
CLINTON TOWNSHIP, MI

HACK

"Boil eggs with ease: add 1 teaspoon of baking soda to water. It will make the shell come off effortlessly."

♥

—CHARLOTTE SHAFFER,
EAST EARL, PA

HACK  87

♥

"Want to know how fresh your eggs are?
Put them in about 4 inches of water. If
they stay on the bottom, they are fresh. If
one end tips up, it is not fresh, use it soon.
If it floats to the top, it has gone bad."

♥

—JUDITH MANOS, WEST ISLIP, NY

HACK 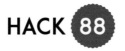 88

♥

"Freeze grapes to chill white wine without watering it down."

♥

—CHARLOTTE SHAFFER, EAST EARL, PA

HACK 89

♥

"Whenever you're having a party and you're serving some type of sangria or large drink, take the juice from the drink and make ice blocks in the freezer. Instead of using ice cubes, the ice block of juice will melt into your drink without watering it down."

♥

—DEB DEBARTOLO, LINCROFT, NY

HACK  90

♥

"When my kiddos were little and just starting solid foods, instead of using a knife to cut up everything, I used scissors— on everything! This makes getting multiple plates ready so much easier."

♥

—JOLEY GREEN, NEWALLA, OK

HACK

♥

"Use a pizza cutter for pancakes, French toast, cutting sandwiches, tiny bite-sized pieces for pizza, whatever your kids eat. It's fast so you'll save yourself time and the struggle of a fork and knife!"

♥

—LINDSAY GOTTHELF, DOUGLASSVILLE, PA

HACK 92

♥

"I keep my spices in a drawer in my pantry. I used to always pick up lots of bottles before I found the right one. Now I label the jars on the lids so I can easily read which spice it is without picking it up."

♥

—Lynette Brenneman, Lancaster, PA

HACK  93

♥

"Make your own spice mixes for
tacos, ranch dressing, and homemade
hamburger helpers in bulk. It's cheaper,
and you control the ingredients!"

♥

—JACKIE FITCH, BURLINGTON, WI

HACK  94

♥

"We usually keep the butter out
in a butter dish. If we run out and
someone wants butter on their bread,
I use a vegetable peeler across the
top of the hard butter to get thin pieces to
put on the bread. Works great,
and the bread doesn't rip."

♥

—Liz Both, Menomonee Falls, WI

HACK 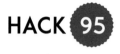 95

♥

"Always keep candy sprinkles in stock! A few sprinkles on just about anything (cottage cheese, fruit, yogurt) can make healthier food look like dessert! Great for picky eaters and mad/sad days! Seasonal sprinkles are a special touch!"

♥

—Paula Arnold, Morrisdale, PA

HACK 96

♥

"To keep a cutting board from sliding on a countertop, cut a piece of leftover rug matting and put under the board. No more slipping!"

♥

—Barbara Nolan, Pleasant Valley, NY

HACK

♥

"If you peel the paper from a traditional American thread spool (Coats & Clark), you will find an attractive 'flower.' This is great to use for pressing cookies such as peanut butter."

♥

—Barbara Shie,
Colorado Springs, CO

HACK 98

♥

"When I make a meal for a large group of guests, I make a note on each recipe of how much I made and how many people it fed. It makes it a little easier the next time!"

♥

—MELISSA WENGER, DALTON, OH

HACK 99

"I put peanut butter into mini condiment squeeze bottles to make it easy and (almost) mess free for kids to put peanut butter on banana and apple slices."

—MELISSA WENGER, DALTON, OH

HACK

♥

"Before cooking a big holiday meal, I sprinkle baking soda over my stovetop. The spills and runovers turn into their own cleanser. After the holiday cooking is done, I take a paintbrush and sweep up any loose baking soda, vacuum it up, or pour vinegar and wipe it up. My teenagers are learning to cook and I have been cleaning and reapplying a lot lately."

♥

—Jackie Kochenower,
New Iberia, LA

HACK

♥

"I taped a list of about thirty-five supper ideas on the inside of a cupboard door. If I have no idea what to make for supper, I can check the list. I got this idea from my friend, Heidi."

♥

—Lynette Brenneman, Lancaster, PA

CLEANING, ORGANIZATION, AND DIY HACKS

♥

This chapter is going to make your life SO much easier! We've got hacks from moms on how to organize your household, how to get your kids to help you clean, how to make cleaning easier for you AND your kids, and even a few tips on some do-it-yourself projects.

HACK 102

♥

"One way to make sure that cleaning jobs don't get missed is to make an itemized list of cleaning jobs by location. As you complete a job, cross it off the list. This also helps if you get interrupted, as you'll know exactly what was or wasn't cleaned. If there are some jobs that kids can do, make a separate list for them and let them cross off the jobs after they are done. Kids love to see that they are accomplishing work like an adult and it gives them a sense of accomplishment."

♥

—ANITA TROYER, FAIRVIEW, MI

HACK 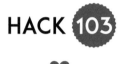 103

♥

"I type a list of things that need cleaned in my house. I tape the paper on the inside of a cupboard door. When I complete something on the list, I check it off until I get to it the next time. Things that do not need cleaned regularly are particularly important to include on the list so I don't forget to do them."

♥

—LYNETTE BRENNEMAN, LANCASTER, PA

HACK

♥

"Our kids all have daily chores. Before school, they need to wipe down the bathroom and kitchen table. After dinner, they need to clean up the kitchen, dining room, bathrooms, living room, and their own rooms. It helps keep the house cleaner and makes them take responsibility for the house."

♥

—HEATHER S., KANSAS CITY, KS

HACK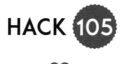

♥

"Introduce your kids to chores early
in their lives. Show them that we all
work as a team and that they can help.
Young kids can help, too."

♥

—Jill Kovach, Cumming, GA

HACK  106

♥

"After supper, my children each do a job in the kitchen. Usually they each use a Norwex cloth to clean and shine one or two kitchen cupboards. I got this idea from my friend Emily."

♥

—LYNETTE BRENNEMAN, LANCASTER, PA

HACK 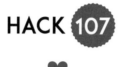 107

♥

"One week I focus my cleaning on the bathrooms and kitchen. The next week I focus on the bedrooms and living room."

♥

—JENNIFER FREED,
HARRISONBURG, VA

HACK

♥

"Use Norwex microfiber and your kids can help (wiping counters, dusting, mopping). Show them how simple it is and send them off for a little teamwork."

♥

—VICKIE ZOLLER, TROY, MI

HACK 109

"Take duct tape and have the kids decorate the lawn bags, both paper and plastic, with Halloween faces. Not only will they help you pick up the leaves, but they become cost-effective masterpieces as well as decorations for your front yard! The kids will take great pride in them, too!"

—MARY LADD, LAKE ORION, MI

HACKS 110-112

SUPERMOM SUGGESTIONS!

Michele Ruvola, Vestal, NY

"Cut citrus fruit in half and use the cut side with salt to scrub stubborn soap and grease scum in tubs and sinks. (Lemons, oranges, or grapefruits)."

♥

"After you've used citrus, when you're done with the peels, throw them down the garbage disposal and turn on to clean and deodorize the garbage disposal."

♥

"Use dryer sheets to clean the slats in blinds, air duct vents, exhaust fans, fan blades, or baseboards."

HACK

♥

"When you are ready to run the dishwasher, hang the dishcloth over the top rack in the front to not have stinky dishcloths anymore."

♥

—Lois Richmond, Hillsgrove, PA

HACK

♥

"Spray your shower and sink down
with the cleaner of your choice and
then take a Magic Eraser and scrub.
Rinse with water and you are finished.
Makes cleaning so much easier!"

♥

—ANGELA DIEM, DENMARK, SC

HACK  115

♥

"Get the children to clean the bathroom every day. It keeps the grossness down."

♥

—JOY REIFF, MOUNT JOY, PA

HACK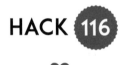

♥

"Shower gel only! Life is too short
to deal with soap scum!"

♥

—Carolyn Dougharty,
San Diego, CA

HACK

♥

"Have the kids strap mop pads on their shoes and have a dance party! The floors will be mopped and shined and everyone will have a good time!"

♥

—MARY LADD, LAKE ORION, MI

HACK

♥

"Add essential oil to your vacuum filter to make the house smell good!!"

♥

—Cathy McIntosh,
Chesterfield Township, MI

HACK  119

♥

"Newspaper cleans glass better than anything you can buy!"

♥

—MARY LADD, LAKE ORION, MI

HACK

"To remove permanent marker from dry-erase surfaces, go over the permanent marker writing with a dry-erase marker, then wipe off with a dry cloth!"

—TRACY GOSSOO, NAPLES, NY

HACK

♥

"To dust the cracks in ornate
furniture, use a Q-tip."

♥

—MARY LADD, LAKE ORION, MI

HACK

♥

"Two hampers (per person): one for underwear, socks, and PJ's . . . and the other for regular clothes. This has saved TONS of time when it comes to sorting wash. And it also saves time with the put away!"

♥

—CATHY MCINTOSH,
CHESTERFIELD TOWNSHIP, MI

HACK 123

♥

"Cut your laundry time by streamlining your routine. I no longer separate clothes by type (whites, colors, etc.). I put each person's clothes in the wash all together as one or two loads, only pulling out the bleach-load clothes. They go from hamper to washer to dryer, back into the hamper (or laundry basket if you feel your hamper is 'dirty') and back to the person to put away. I cut out sorting and folding time, which added at least two hours to my laundry time each week. I only have to sort socks and underwear as one load."

♥

—BRENDA SCHNARRS,
CLINTON TOWNSHIP, MI

HACK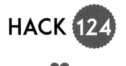

♥

"I assigned each child their own 'laundry day.' One-on-one, that child and I would sort, wash, dry, and fold JUST their laundry (they put them away). In a very short time and at a young age, they could do their own laundry and took pride in doing so, freeing up my time for other household duties."

♥

—AVONELLE SOLLARS, ALBANY, OH

HACK

♥

"Each child has their own laundry basket and when it gets full, I just dump that whole basket in except towels and church clothes."

♥

—JOY REIFF, MOUNT JOY, PA

HACK

♥

"Sort and hang each family member's laundry separately on the wash line. This makes folding wash a breeze because it's all sorted already."

♥

—Joy Martin, Richland, PA

HACK  127

♥

"If things seem overwhelming, do one load of laundry from start to finish a day."

♥

—JENNIFER FREED,
HARRISONBURG, VA

HACK 128

♥

"Cool children's food down faster by getting a bowl of ice and putting their dish on top for a few minutes."

♥

—MARY LADD, LAKE ORION, MI

HACK 129

♥

"Put a paper towel at the bottom of
the lunch pail. If something spills, it is
easier to clean out the lunch pail."

♥

—CAROL EVELETH, CHEYENNE, WY

HACK

♥

"Put a cupcake paper in your car's drink holder. When it starts to get yucky, throw it out and replace."

♥

—BARBARA SHIE,
COLORADO SPRINGS, CO

HACK  131

♥

"If you lost a small item, put a nylon knee-high over the end of your vacuum wand. Vacuum the area where you think your lost item is and hopefully it will be found on the end of your vacuum."

♥

—CAROL EVELETH, CHEYENNE, WY

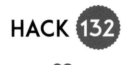

♥

"Have a place for everything.
Make sure all household members
know where things go."

♥

—JENNIFER FREED,
HARRISONBURG, VA

HACKS 133–135

SUPERMOM SUGGESTIONS!

Lynette Brenneman, Lancaster, PA

"I learned this tip from my friend, Heather. I keep a decorative basket on top of the dryer. I put things that need to be returned to others in the basket. Then, when I'm going to see that person, I know where the item is."

♥

"When I put a can on my pantry shelf, I sometimes use a Sharpie marker to write the expiration date on top of the can so I can quickly see when something is about to expire."

♥

"I bought a clear plastic makeup organizer for the bathroom closet. It has thin compartments (maybe for lipstick) that our electric toothbrushes fit into perfectly. Now they stand up straight instead of laying around on the shelf."

HACK 136

♥

"Use a car seatback organizer or shoe organizer that hangs on a door and use it in the bathroom. Hang it over the bathroom door and use the pockets to organize baby shampoo, baby lotion, diaper cream, extra diapers, those tiny hooded bath towels, tiny baby washcloths, and even little tiny socks/tights. The more pockets, the more you can store in there. As the baby grows, you can change out some of the items for favorite bath toy storage and even the little underwear when potty training. It keeps everything together that you could need in the bathroom for baby/toddler use."

♥

—TINA KASSA, HEWITT, TX

HACK  137

♥

"When using a large roll of tape
or duct tape, put a paperclip on the
just cut end, so it will be easy to find the
end next time you use the roll."

♥

—BARBARA SHIE,
COLORADO SPRINGS, CO

HACK

♥

"Store cupcake liners in a mason jar.
Makes the jar look pretty and you can
eliminate cupcake packaging that takes
up precious room in your cabinets."

♥

—MICHELE RUVOLA, VESTAL, NY

HACK 139

♥

"Instead of using a drawer or cabinet
when space is limited, use your trivets
and odd dishes to make a wall special.
When you need them, they are handy, but
meanwhile, they'll decorate your wall!"

♥

—MARY LADD, LAKE ORION, MI

HACK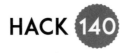

♥

"Magazine holders are the perfect size to stack baking pans to keep them organized in your cabinets."

♥

—MICHELE RUVOLA, VESTAL, NY

HACK

♥

"To keep large bowl and Tupperware
lids organized, I put two mini tension
rods vertically in the cupboard about
four inches from the side of the cupboard.
The lids stand upright and it is easy
to find the one I need."

♥

—Melissa Wenger, Dalton, OH

HACK  142

♥

"If you have an upstairs or basement, place a basket on the stairs and fill with things that need to go up or down. Then you can make one trip instead of lots of trips."

♥

—JENNIFER FREED, HARRISONBURG, VA

HACK

♥

"I keep my recipes cards in a photo album with 4 × 6 pockets. At the beginning of each section, I put a card with recipes listed that are in cookbooks and their page number."

♥

—MELISSA WENGER, DALTON, OH

HACK

♥

"Reuse last year's numerous refrigerator art for the covers of your photo albums so you can keep the treasures."

♥

—Mary Ladd, Lake Orion, MI

HACK

♥

"Cut up old T-shirts, towels, and even socks and use them for rags to clean with and toss in the washer when finished. This saves on paper towels!"

♥

—Angela Diem, Denmark, SC

HACK

♥

"If your coffee is taking longer to brew than usual, put white vinegar in the water reservoir and brew several cycles of vinegar. Then brew just regular water several times."

♥

—CAROL EVELETH, CHEYENNE, WY

HACK

♥

"Old, broken jewelry makes great
bling for any project!"

♥

—MARY LADD, LAKE ORION, MI

HACK 148

♥

"Toilet backed up? No plunger? Use liquid hand soap—dump some in the toilet, wait five minutes, and flush again. Clears the clog."

♥

—Judith Manos, West Islip, NY

HACK 149

♥

"Gather scraps of old bar soap equal to 4 ounces, which is the weight of a regular bar of soap. Shred the soap using a cheese grater or a potato peeler. Heat the soap pieces in a pot with approximately 8 to 9 cups of water until it melts. Use less water if you want to make a creamy body wash instead of liquid hand soap. This is just optional, but you can add 1 tablespoon of vegetable glycerin, which will help moisturize the skin. Remove melted soap from the heat and let it sit covered for 12 to 24 hours. After the soap thickens overnight, use a whisk or a mixer to blend it together. If it's too thick or too thin, you can make adjustments and repeat the previous steps as necessary. Transfer to containers for storage."

♥

—CAROL EVELETH, CHEYENNE, WY

HACK  150

♥

"How to caulk like a pro: Use painter's tape just above and just below where you want the caulk to go. Make sure to keep the same gap size the entire length of your project. Squeeze a thick line of caulk between the pieces of tape. Run a finger across the caulk to smooth it out. Wait about five to ten minutes and peel up the painters tape. End result will be beautiful, crisp, clean caulk lines."

♥

—JUDITH MANOS, WEST ISLIP, NY

HACKS 151–153

SUPERMOM SUGGESTIONS!

Mary Ladd, Lake Orion, MI

"Remnants of wallpaper or wrapping paper make great backdrops when framing pictures."

♥

"Cover a plain lampshade with material to make it exactly what you want/need!"

♥

"Scratches on top of a coffee table? Take a piece of material, cover to the size of your table, and add a piece of plexiglass on top."

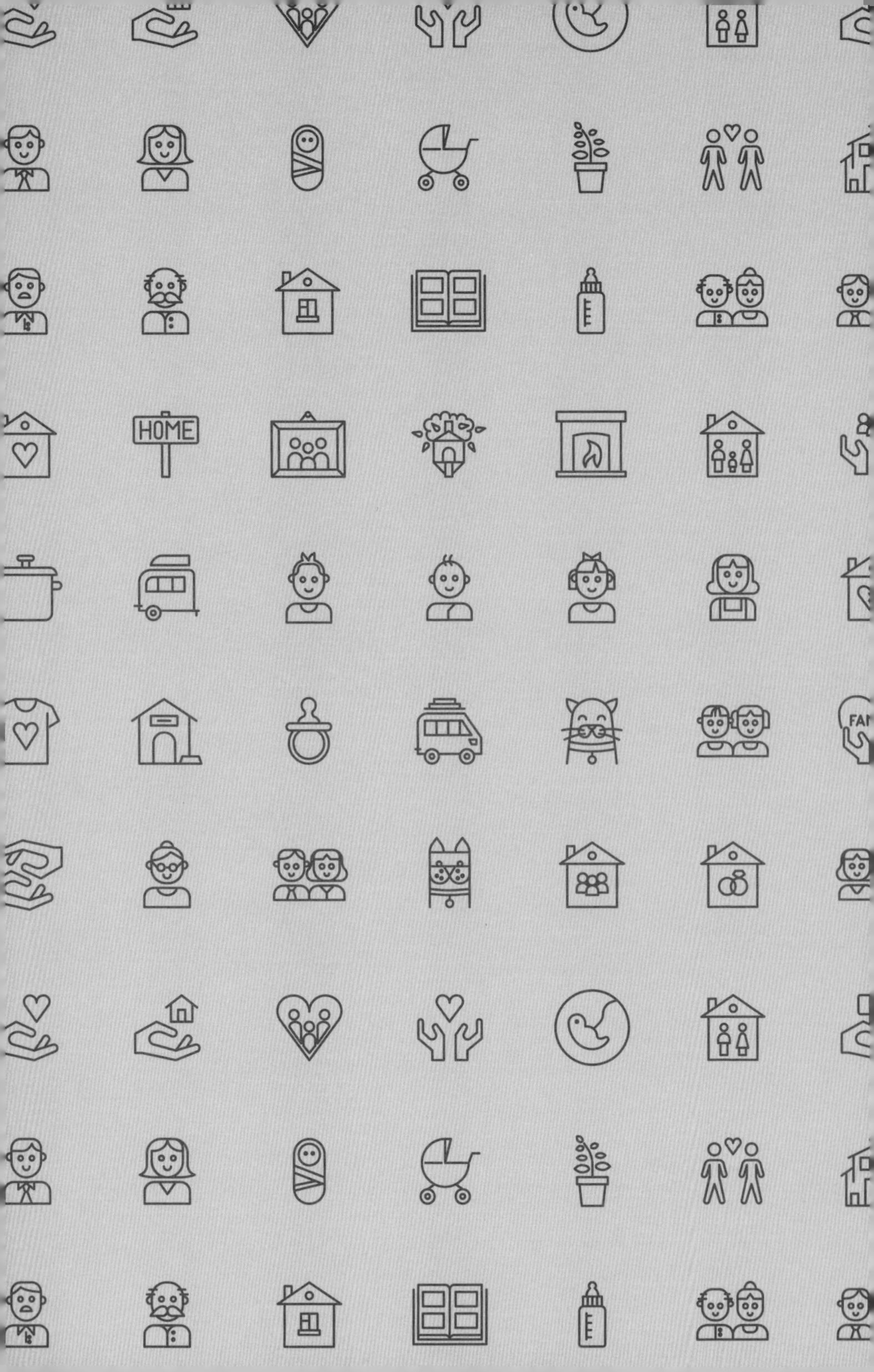
HOME

SHOPPING AND GIFTING HACKS

♥

Do you ever wonder how your friends ALWAYS find the best deals? Are you always running to the store for more gift bags or wrapping paper for your kids' friends birthday parties? This chapter will help you conquer the shopping and the gifting in your life.

HACK 154

♥

"You can leverage your store's loyalty card to get the most out of your back-to-school or holiday shopping. Some stores will offer fuel rewards for gift card purchases, up to 4× the fuel points. If you watch their sales, and load their digital coupons for these incentives, you can get money off a gift card purchase AND save a huge amount of money on gas. I started watching more closely this summer and have had at least $1 off per gallon for nearly every fill-up. Our back-to-school shopping was SO much easier because the cost didn't seem so painful when paying for it a little bit at a time."

♥

—LUANN EDWARDS,
WILMINGTON, OH

HACK

"I keep my shopping list on my phone. Every time I think of something I need, I add it to the list. This way I don't lose or forget the list. Some grocery store apps even have built-in shopping lists."

—LYNETTE BRENNEMAN, LANCASTER, PA

HACK

♥

"Keep reusable shopping bags in your car. I use them at Aldi, but then end up being able to use them to keep the kids' random objects in when they come home from a party, etc. The key is to remember to put them back in your car right away after they're unpacked. I always keep one cooler shopping bag in my car as well for frozen goods."

♥

—HOPE COMERFORD, CLINTON TOWNSHIP, MI

HACK

♥

"Use a 'D' ring/carabiner to hold your reuseable shopping bags. I hook them on the grate in the front of the baby seat. That way they don't take up any room in my shopping basket."

♥

—BARBARA SHIE,
COLORADO SPRINGS, CO

HACK

♥

"When shopping, have a big bag or cooler in the trunk of your car and load your groceries directly into it. Then when you get home, all you have to do is carry it into the house. Keeps loose groceries, etc., much more contained!"

♥

—ANGELA DIEM, DENMARK, SC

HACK  159

♥

"If needing to save money and brand names are your child's 'thing,' go to Salvation Army, find the brand of jeans in any size, and add the label to a favorite, more affordable, pair of jeans that fit!"

♥

—MARY LADD, LAKE ORION, MI

HACK  160

♥

"Because I'm a bargain shopper, I like to buy gifts for birthdays and Christmas whenever I see a sale. Then I keep a list of what I buy for people so that I don't double buy. Whenever I hear family talking about things they want to get someday, I write those down, and if I see a good sale, I get those things. By doing this, I spread the Christmas spending over the entire year and I don't have to face the big shopping crowds in December."

♥

—ANITA TROYER, FAIRVIEW, MI

HACK 161

♥

"Pick a theme gift for each year that you can use for everyone—family, friends, teachers. Homemade soaps/ lotions, fun socks, blankets, gloves, etc. You can watch for a great sale and still personalize it to each person with an easy variation on your theme."

♥

—Jackie Fitch, Burlington, WI

HACK  162

♥

"Iron colored leaves between wax paper to use as wrapping paper for cookies or candy."

♥

—MARY LADD, LAKE ORION, MI

HACK

♥

"I only buy solid white wrapping paper. I collect all colors of bows. No matter what the event, I have the appropriate gift wrap."

♥

—LYNN INVERSO, WARRINGTON, PA

HACKS 164–166

SUPERMOM SUGGESTIONS!

Natalie Trombley, Rochester Hills, MI

"Keep a stash of neutral brown gift bags along with different colors of tissue paper."

♥

"Buy Scotch tape during after-Christmas sales to get them on sale."

♥

"Buy bulk blank greeting cards and have kids 'create' their own cards for family/ friends' birthdays, etc."

HACK

♥

"Recently we have made our birthday gifts for siblings and parents be a meal out. That way we get to spend time with family members and nobody really needs anything."

♥

—JENNIFER FREED, HARRISONBURG, VA

HACK 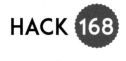 168

♥

"Put an empty toilet paper roll
over a roll of wrapping paper to
keep it from unrolling."

♥

—CHARLOTTE SHAFFER,
EAST EARL, PA

TRAVELING HACKS

♥

Traveling with kids can be down-right exhausting! Just thinking about packing is enough to make some decide to stay home. We've got lots of hacks in this chapter from moms who really know how to make traveling easier . . . whether it's for a big trip, or even just in the car for day-to-day errand running!

HACK

♥

"I grew up playing the alphabet game in the car! It really makes the time go by faster. You'll start with the letter 'A.' Whoever sees a sign with the letter 'A' first gets a point. You have to do the letters in order, so, 'B' must be found next and so on. You can keep points with fingers and toes, or mom and dad can keep score for the kiddos."

♥

—HOPE COMERFORD,
CLINTON TOWNSHIP, MI

HACK

♥

"Keep an 'on-the-go' bag in the car. Fill with playing cards, mini figurines, mini puzzles, notebooks, pencils/ crayons. (Lots of these I kept from birthday party favors.) Simple things to keep kids occupied when waiting somewhere or at restaurants."

♥

—NATALIE TROMBLEY, ROCHESTER HILLS, MI

HACK  171

♥

"Have kids that get carsick? Always bring an ice cream bucket with a lid. Line it with grocery bags, keep more on hand in the seatback storage. When your kid gets sick in the bucket, just tie the bag up and dispose! No more messes in the car seats!"

♥

—JOLEY GREEN, NEWALLA, OK

HACK

♥

"Before a trip, sit down with the kids and make a list of things they need to pack. Have them check the items off the list as they pack. It gives them independence and you a bit more free time, plus results in fewer arguments and teaches your children how to pack in the future."

♥

—HOPE COMERFORD,
CLINTON TOWNSHIP, MI

HACK 173

♥

"When traveling with little ones, I pack everything needed for an outfit in a gallon-sized Ziploc bag. Whoever is helping get the kiddo ready in the morning only needs to grab a bag or the kids can grab a bag and get ready themselves. We then have a bag for anything that gets overly soiled if needed."

♥

—SHANI BELL, PHOENIX, AZ

HACK

♥

"When traveling, pack each item in a plastic Ziploc bag according to type. Then when you need to find something in the bottom of the suitcase, you won't get your clothing dirty or messed up by removing from the suitcase. Also, if a liquid leaks, it won't make a mess on your clothing."

♥

—ANITA TROYER, FAIRVIEW, MI

HACK

♥

"When packing for your family,
pack each day's clothes in a large
Ziploc bag. Label each bag with the
day the clothes will be worn. Easy and
quick dressing so you can get out
of your hotel and on with your fun!"

♥

—JACKIE FITCH, BURLINGTON, WI

HACK  176

"Roll the clothes and pack an empty spray bottle. You can get a full week of clothes in a carry on!! When you get to your hotel, ask for extra hangers at the front desk and hang your clothes, give them a spritz of water, and let the wrinkles hang out. In less than an hour, your clothes will be unwrinkled and ready to go. If you are in a hurry to change, spritz and use the blow dryer to dry the clothes. It's faster than ironing them."

—LAURA BRUEDELE, CEDARBURG, WI

HACK

♥

"If you travel internationally, there are some things you should always do:

1. Travel with a water bottle, as you never know when you will be at a location where you have access to water.
2. Always ask if tap water is safe to drink.
3. Always travel with some small American currency to tip natives who may carry your bags.
4. Always carry some snacks, as eating schedules may not be predictable.
5. Read about the country you are planning to visit. If you are buying souvenirs, what might be available? Are there cultural do's or don'ts?"

♥

—ANITA TROYER, FAIRVIEW, MI

HACK  178

♥

"Make sure you always take a picture of your luggage before traveling. This will help speed the paperwork process if your luggage is lost or damaged."

♥

—Judith Manos, West Islip, NY

HACK  179

"Always have plasticware wrapped in napkins when traveling. It makes it much easier than trying to carry them all separately."

—MARY LADD, LAKE ORION, MI

HEALTH AND FITNESS HACKS

♥

Moms need to take care of their littles AND themselves! That's where this chapter comes in. We've got hacks for new moms, moms-to-be, and seasoned moms to keep you all healthy and fit.

HACK 180

♥

"Keep a list of doctors, medications, and allergies behind your driver's license. In an emergency, you want the ER to contact your doctor if possible. If your child has special needs or medications, keep it on the list, too. You can also have small pictures on the list with family members' names. When I was nine, six of us were in a horrible accident and I was the only one without a head injury."

♥

—JEAN HANSEN, BELTSVILLE, MD

HACK  181

♥

"As a mom of four, I taught the kids to gargle with diluted salt water—½ teaspoon table salt in 4 ounces water—every time they went to the bathroom. We avoided strep throat and kept the kids in school!"

♥

—Jean Hansen, Beltsville, MD

HACK

♥

"If you have trouble with constipation from a low-carb diet, or to help with a high-stress life, take a daily dose of Natural Calm, a magnesium supplement (preferably the magnesium with calcium blend), for a better night's sleep."

♥

—CAROL EVELETH, CHEYENNE, WY

HACK

♥

"We don't all have time, patience, pain tolerance, or money to do the bikini wax thing. I use Young Living Tea Tree essential oil on the bikini line to reduce red bumps, itching, and irritation from shaving when I can't make it to the salon. Immediate relief!"

♥

—GRETCHEN MACARTHUR, TRAVERSE CITY, MI

HACK

♥

"For new moms: if you prepare your breasts for breastfeeding ahead of time, you will have greater success. Use a washcloth each day on your nipples to toughen them up."

♥

—Mary Ladd, Lake Orion, MI

HACK

♥

"For the postpartum mom: you can make an ice pack for the perineal area by saturating a baby diaper and putting it in the freezer. Once it's frozen or slushy, put the diaper in your underwear for cooling relief. It also absorbs the blood. This is an old-school nursing hack that unfortunately we're not allowed to use at the hospital anymore because clean diapers in the freezer are 'unsanitary.'"

♥

—ANDREA VRBA, SAN ANTONIO, CA

HACK

♥

"Feminine napkins cut in half work better and cheaper than breastfeeding pads."

♥

—MARY LADD, LAKE ORION, MI

HACK  187

♥

"For a better night of sleep, make a small 9 × 9 pillow and fill with dried hops, lavender, and chamomile. Slip the small herb pillow under the pillowcase on your regular pillow and let the relaxing aroma induce a good night's sleep."

♥

—CAROL EVELETH, CHEYENNE, WY

HACK  188

♥

"Always feel tired even after getting a good, long sleep? You are probably dehydrated. Drink some water immediately when you wake up."

♥

—JUDITH MANOS, WEST ISLIP, NY

HACK  189

♥

"I am hypoglycemic, so it's important that I have a healthy start to my day as well as healthy snacks. To get a good start to the day, I like to have protein but lack the time required each morning to fry an egg, so I fry them ahead of time and freeze them. It is easy to reheat them each morning and make a breakfast sandwich. I often have fried sausage or bacon to also put into my sandwich. For a healthy snack, I make my own snack mix and put into Ziploc bags. Make the mix to suit your taste, but some suggestions are: peanuts, sesame sticks, M&M's, raisins or Craisins, chocolate chips, etc."

♥

—ANITA TROYER, FAIRVIEW, MI

HACK  190

♥

"To get night vision, keep one eye closed in the well-lit area, then open it in the darkness; that eye will be able to see in the dark. This is why pirates wore eye patches."

♥

—Judith Manos, West Islip, NY

HACK 191

♥

"Working out doesn't have to happen in the gym. Let your kids be your trainer! Set out for a walk with your kids and let their imaginations pave the way. Let them give you fun and different ways to move along your walk. Maybe they want you to skip, or walk with your hands waving over your head, shuffle your feet from side to side, or hop like a bunny. Let them get as creative and silly as they want. You'll get in a great workout and you'll all have a fun and memorable time together as a family!"

♥

—HOPE COMERFORD,
CLINTON TOWNSHIP, MI

HACK

♥

"Do your kids like to play Simon Says?
Instead of playing regular Simon Says,
play Fitness Simon Says, which only
varies from the original version in that
all actions have to be fitness related. You
can start and set the example, or you
can let the kids start. Either way, you'll
all be having fun and getting in a great
workout while you do it!"

♥

—HOPE COMERFORD,
CLINTON TOWNSHIP, MI

HACK

♥

"Park in the back of the parking lot when shopping. It can help get in your steps for the day."

♥

—HEATHER S., KANSAS CITY, KS

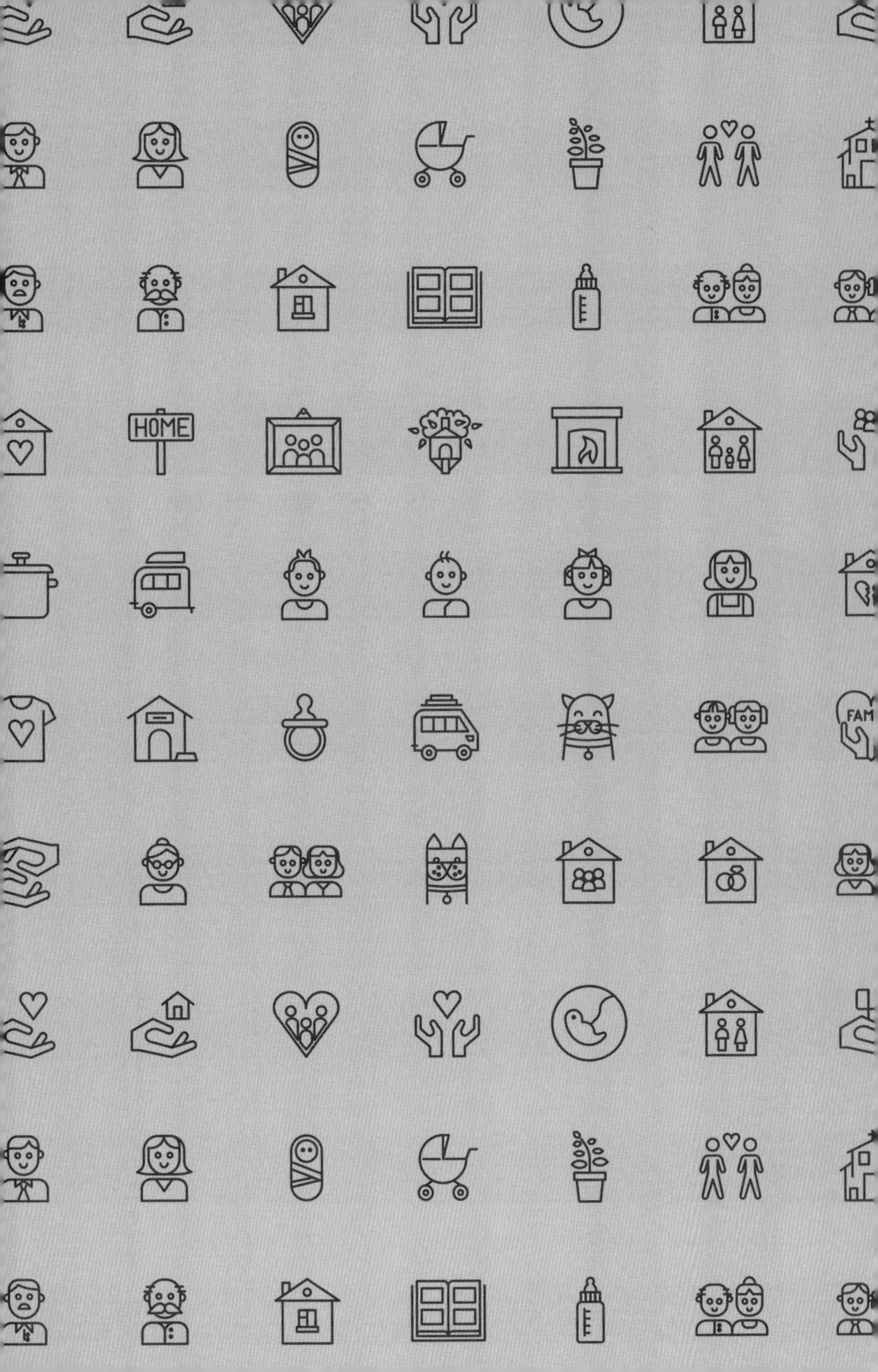
HOME
FAM

ADDITIONAL HELPFUL HACKS

♥

Since you're a mom, you know that not everything fits into a tiny, neat box. Here you'll find some helpful hacks for other areas of your life.

HACK

♥

"Waterproof mascara is great for the water, but kind of a pain to get off. Instead of using expensive waterproof eye makeup remover, use good ol' coconut oil to remove it instead. That's right! The kind you cook with! Use a cotton ball or cotton round and a small amount of coconut oil, and gently wipe the waterproof mascara away!"

♥

—HOPE COMERFORD,
CLINTON TOWNSHIP, MI

HACK 195

♥

"Rinse your hair with lemon juice.
It brightens up blond hair and
brings out the highlights."

♥

—MARY LADD, LAKE ORION, MI

HACK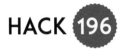

"Put cinnamon in cracks on counters and cupboards to keep ants out."

—Joy Reiff, Mount Joy, PA

HACK  197

"Rub a walnut on damaged wooden
furniture to cover up dings."

—CHARLOTTE SHAFFER,
EAST EARL, PA

HACK 198

♥

"Want your carved pumpkin to last longer? Apply some petroleum jelly to the cuts. This will extend your pumpkin's life."

♥

—JUDITH MANOS, WEST ISLIP, NY

HACK 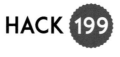 199

"Have a ring stuck on your finger? Don't struggle with soap or cut the ring off. Spray Windex on it and it will slip right off. A jewelry store owner told me about this trick and it works like a charm."

—JOCELYN RAYMOND,
PERTH, ONTARIO, CANADA

HACK

♥

"This is for people who paint or craft. I take the foam trays that meat comes on and wash them with soap and hot water. Once clean, they are great to use for painting small crafts. They clean off nicely. When they get old, throw them away."

♥

—SALLY TREDINNICK, WILKES-BARRE, PA

HACK  201

♥

"Want your whole bathroom to match?
Shower curtains make great drapes, too!"

♥

—MARY LADD, LAKE ORION, MI

HACK

♥

"To keep all your computer passwords in one place, get a small (5 × 8) address book to use. Place the company alphabetically in ink, and then just put "U" for user name, and "P" for password (in pencil). I also add the date in pencil."

♥

—Barbara Shie,
Colorado Springs, CO

HACK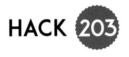

♥

"When Googling a computer error, add 'solved' to search query to find answer much faster. 'Error _____ solved.'"

♥

—JUDITH MANOS, WEST ISLIP, NY

HACK

♥

"When using your iPhone calculator, swipe left or right in the calculation field to delete the last digit, so you don't have to start over."

♥

—Judith Manos, West Islip, NY

ABOUT THE AUTHOR

♥

Hope Comerford is a mom, wife, elementary school music teacher, blogger, recipe developer, public speaker, ALM Zone Fitness Motivator, Young Living Essential Oils enthusiast/ educator, and published author.

In 2010, Hope started her blog, *A Busy Mom's Slow Cooker Adventures* to simply share the recipes she was making with her family and friends. She never imagined people all over the world would begin visiting her page and sharing her recipes with others as well. In 2013, Hope self-published her first cookbook *Slow Cooker Recipes: 10 Ingredients or Less and Gluten-Free* and then later wrote *The Gluten-Free Slow Cooker.*

Hope has written many books, including *Fix-It and Forget-It Lazy & Slow Cookbook, Fix-It and Forget-It Healthy Slow Cooker Cookbook, Fix-It and Forget-It Favorite Slow Cooker Recipes for Mom, Fix-It and Forget-It Favorite Slow Cooker Recipes for Dad,* and *Fix-It and Forget-It Instant Pot Cookbook.*

Hope lives in the city of Clinton Township, Michigan, near Metro Detroit and is a Michigan native. She has been happily married to her husband and best friend, Justin, since 2008. Together they have two children, Ella and Gavin, who are her motivation, inspiration, and heart. In her spare time, Hope enjoys traveling, singing, cooking, reading books, spending time with friends and family, and relaxing.